You Want Me to What?

An Odyssey of a Reluctant Primary Personal Caregiver for a Double-Lung Transplant Patient

Donna M. Mogan, PhD

Copyright © 2018 DONNA MOGAN. All rights reserved. No portion of this book may be reproduced mechanically, electronically, or by any other means, including photocopying, without written permission of the publisher. It is illegal to copy this book, post it to a website, or distribute it by any other means without permission from the publisher.

Limits of Liability and Disclaimer of Warranty
The author and publisher shall not be liable for your misuse of this material. This book is strictly for informational and educational purposes.

Warning – Disclaimer
The purpose of this book is to educate and entertain. The author and/or publisher do not guarantee that anyone following these techniques, suggestions, tips, ideas, or strategies will become successful. The author and/or publisher shall have neither liability nor responsibility to anyone with respect to any loss or damage caused, or alleged to be caused, directly or indirectly, by the information contained in this book.

ISBN: 9781723711749

Contents

Introduction 5

Chapter 1: How Did This Happen? 11
The Surprise That Came from out of the Blue

Chapter 2: How Did I Get This Job? 21
This Wasn't on My Resume

Chapter 3: Where Am I Going and How Do
I Get There? 33
The Maze of Mania

Chapter 4: Is This the Yellow Brick Road? 47
Where Are the Munchkins?

Chapter 5: How Much Did You Say That
Would Cost? 61
You're Kidding, Right?

Chapter 6: Where Do We Go Now for This
Transplant? 69
The Bricks Are Pretty Dusty

Chapter 7: Is the Wizard of Oz Available? 79
A Heart, a Brain and Courage

Chapter 8: What Happens Once the Ruby Slippers
Have Been Clicked? 93

Chapter 9: Are We There Yet? 103
The Wicked Witch Is Dead

Epilogue: Is That a Rainbow? 111

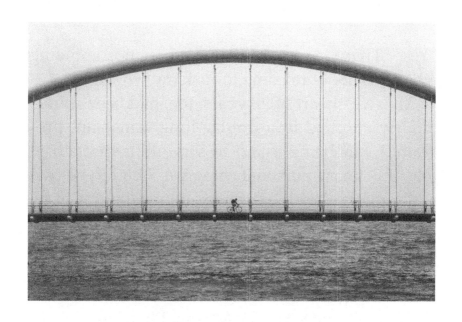

Introduction

"Diseases can be our spiritual flat tires—disruptions in our lives that seem to be disasters at the time but end by redirecting our lives in a meaningful way."
~Bernie S. Siegel

DO YOU FEEL LIKE you would describe yourself as an older, wiser, well-educated and seasoned individual with strength of character? Have you faced a number of serious traumatic or challenging situations throughout your life? Do you feel you can reason and problem solve with above-average credibility?

When asked these questions several years ago, I would have calmly answered with confidence,

"Yes." That was too glib an answer not knowing what was about to come to rock my world.

My sweetheart of 20 years, Joe, had been miraculously enrolled in a double-lung transplant program. I was being asked to serve in a specialized role of primary personal caregiver. I had to be part of this journey with him every step of the way as he was being prepared for this complex life or death procedure. My odyssey along this road had me feeling like Dorothy in *The Wizard of Oz* as she entered into a strange land.

My name is Donna M. Mogan, PhD. I am a Consulting Psychologist and a Transformational Personal and Professional Life Coach. For many years I have helped my clients reach effective and efficient solutions when they faced stressful challenges. My belief is that each transition is meant to give a person a more expanded understanding of who they really are. This can lead to better choices with ongoing life adventures. The struggles often deepen insight into a myriad of hidden capabilities and strengths. With the experience of the last several years I went through a true "doctor heal thyself" challenge.

That being said, I don't know about you, but for me I usually approach my transitions with a lot of kicking and screaming. I can drag my chains of resistance for a pretty good stretch. Like most people, I don't like moving out of my comfort zone. Also like many people, my life has been filled with numerous situations in which this had to occur. Life is filled with these challenges that can lead us into more self-discovery and confidence.

I have added years of education, training and numerous professional credits to my name. However, it has been my personal life experiences of transitions that I value the most. They have been the icing on the cake in relating with the wonderful people I serve professionally as both a coach and consultant.

Though I am now in my "elder wisdom" years, the challenges just keep coming. Yes, I still approach change transitions with grunts and groans as I hang on to my resistance chain, but at least it is not for quite as long as it used to be.

My intent is to share with you the surprises and obstacles on my path with Joe towards his double-lung transplant. I became a specialized primary personal caregiver that increased in intensity with all it entailed. But I also want to assure you that this path, as have all the others, eventually brought me into some wondrous new experiences. I have expanded understandings and insights of myself, Joe, family members, friends and my Creator in ways that were beyond what I had imagined. I have gained a greater and deeper appreciation for the life paths and stories of many others as well as my own.

I do want to provide a "fast forward" qualifier here that gives you the good news: the end of this odyssey is filled with joy. Joe made it successfully through the transplant process, and he is thriving today.

I believe that humans are mixed bags that run the gamut of emotional, psychological, physiological and spiritual characteristics. Every person is unique in how they process their challenges. Yet depending on the situation, similarities among people are also evident. Listening to and reading about others' experiences often gives the insights we need to go through our own. Actually, in all my years of living and working in the areas of personal, professional and spiritual development, I think we are pretty darn fantastic!

I wrote this book for those of you who have found yourselves in the challenging role of being a primary personal caregiver. With new environments, tasks and even your relationships changing, you may often find yourself asking, "You want me to *what?*" You feel incredulous that your life has taken this unfamiliar and unwanted turn. The chapters in this book address some of the issues that you may be facing. I learned a few lessons that I share with you at the end of the chapters. I have also included some exercises/techniques. They may prove helpful in giving you some clarity and comfort as you journey forward.

You may have found that your world has been turned upside down and inside out. Most people will be focusing on the patient. It's not likely that what you are going through will be appreciated by too many others who have not lived through this situation. They may seriously care but cannot fully appreciate it. Let's face it, did you know what this was *really* all about before it happened to you?

The rules of English suggest that we do not capitalize certain words as we write. However, wherever you see "primary personal caregiver," understand that I would prefer to write "Primary Personal Caregiver." I really want to emphasize how important and unique this role is especially when dealing with life and death situations and patients. Within the transplant system I found myself a part of, there is a detailed *Primary Personal Caregiver Guide* with which one has to become quite familiar.

Much information is written about what the transplant patient can expect and thank goodness for that. However, since nobody wants to be thought of as "whiners," not too much is in the marketplace about what the primary personal caregiver's experiences are actually like.

As I describe my personal odyssey from my vantage point, maybe you will relate to what you are experiencing along your own path. As I travelled through the maze I made some new self-discoveries. I found not only self-deceptions and failures but beauty, strengths and triumphs as well. Perhaps you will too.

So here we go...

"Praise the bridge that carried you over."
- George Colman

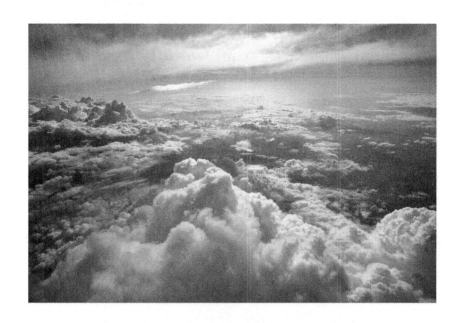

CHAPTER 1:

How Did This Happen?

The Surprise That Came from out of the Blue

"Hope is independent of the apparatus of logic."
-Norman Cousins

BEING AN UNPAID PRIMARY personal caregiver for a family member who in my case is a double-lung transplant patient, is really difficult and, often, thankless. Your worldly environment devolves into oxygen tanks, bi-paps and noisy oxygen concentrators. You probably have wheelchairs, rollators (walkers with wheels) and canes parked here and there. Couches and lounge chairs may have become beds. There are shower chairs now in your bathrooms along with drawers or shelves filled with medications.

Plans for renovations and additions for your home are pretty much out of the picture now. Your place, instead, is functioning and feeling more and more like a rehab center. The main visitors to your home include a nurse, occupational therapist, and the oxygen delivery man. The usual visitors like neighbors and out-of-towners have thinned out.

Your very ill loved one is often trying to balance between trying to stay alive and wanting to die. Their world is bleak and yours is probably getting darker as well.

Allow me, please, to take hold of your hand, embrace you with a big hug, and tell you how I meandered through the maze of mass confusion you have probably been experiencing. Your experience is unique to you as mine has been to me. I believe, however, you will find a number of similarities and correlations encountered along this path to which you can relate.

I have made it through yet another major life event of having my world turned upside down.

There were surprise surgeries, hospital stays, financial changes, home maintenance challenges and relationship shifts among the many obstacles.

The journey has, indeed, been quite a trip. Yet, here I am on the other side of "shadowland" and finally able to appreciate the insights and wisdom gained for my life at this time. As I share this with you my deepest intent is for you to expand your understanding with new insights and appreciation of your own experience.

So, how did I get this job? It began with the chronic condition my partner of 18 years was facing. Joe had COPD (Chronic Obstructive Pulmonary Disease), emphysema, and acute asthma. He was in his mid-60s, and his lungs were dying. He had less than two years of life left.

He had never smoked cigarettes. He did smoke little cigarillos on occasion and a pipe from time to time. However, he had also been surrounded by secondary smoke throughout his life. During his extensive naval career Joe had been exposed to Agent Orange during his Vietnam deployment as well as to toxic asbestos materials used in the ships on which he served. Many former military service people have suffered from these poisonous environments. COPD and lung cancer are common conditions that resulted from their heroic service to our country.

Unbeknown to us, Joe's pulmonologist, a top physician in the field, was working behind the scenes to get him into a lung-transplant program at Duke University Hospital in Durham, North Carolina. The doctor had trained several of the members of the transplant teams. He knew they were the best in the country.

Because of his age, we never thought this was a possibility for Joe. The day arrived when the doctor was able to share with us what he had been doing. I will never forget it. We were in his office on a regular visit, which usually showed how much worse his condition was. The good doctor became real quiet and looked back and forth between us. Then he started to smile. I thought, "Well this is different. How could there have been any improvement? Maybe he is getting ready to tell us he is retiring and is happy about it."

Then, in his somewhat heavy accent he began to tell us about the lung transplant program. It was internationally renowned. I figured he was just about to share how proud he was to have been a major player in working with many of the program's medical teams. Never in our wildest dreams did we expect what he was to say next. The green light had been given for Joe to go to Duke Hospital right away to be evaluated for the program. We knew the doctor would not have set this up if he didn't truly think that Joe had a fighting chance to receive the transplant. Hope that had been long dismissed now came alive.

Chapter 1: How Did This Happen?

We left the office in an unfamiliar state of mind. It had been a long time since we were grinning and chatting away about the future with fun scenarios. Our energy was mixed with awe, hope and a bit of giddiness. Even though it was raining outside, the inside of our car was filling up with sunshine. We didn't really know how this was all going to go down but we did know we would rise to this fantastic opportunity.

"Hope is like a road in the country; there was never a road, but when many people walk on it, the road comes into existence."
~Lin Yutang

Joe and I were living in Virginia. About two weeks after getting the go-ahead from the doctor, we received the scheduled appointments and a large orientation package from Duke Hospital. In it were forms to fill out and lists of recommended places to stay close to the hospital.

We drove to North Carolina for about three and a half hours and were able to stay in a nice hotel near the hospital that offered handicap accommodations. They also offered a discounted rate for people associated with the Duke Hospital transplant programs. After a rest, we drove around the area a little and found our route to the hospital.

The next day we left early to get to the first appointment. We used valet parking so we wouldn't be late by not knowing where we would be going. The hospital is huge. There are miles of corridors and numerous floors to navigate. As I was pushing Joe in his wheelchair, trying to read directories, his own anxiety steadily grew. He would get frustrated with me if we were not at the right place at least ten minutes before that appointment. Thank goodness people were often helpful in giving directions. Strangers were much kinder to me than was Joe. Later, I think I got to the point where I was kinder to strangers than I was to Joe. Though understandable, his stress was always a stress builder for me.

Over the next four days the extensive evaluation took place. This included but was not limited to blood work, pulmonary tests, and nutrition and physical therapy reviews. He also had to be seen by a surgical team, urologist, pulmonologist, cardiologist, sociologist, and psychologist. There were also appointments with a financial advisor and administrator.

One surgeon served as the Dutch uncle as he gravely explained how this would be the most excruciating experience of Joe's life. He was carefully watching both of our reactions as he took us through some of the more lurid details of the actual transplant. The pre-op and post-op scenarios were also pretty strong reality bites.

There were many forms to fill out, including ones for me. One of these was an in-depth questionnaire which outlined what would be expected of me as the Primary Personal Caregiver. I was expected to sign it. I did, but only after taking a deep breath. This was the first inkling I had of how deep this water was that I was wading into.

AT THIS POINT I would like to give you a little scenario about how Joe and I first met.

I was sitting at my computer one October evening surfing the net. It had been three months since I had ended a long-term relationship with someone else. I wasn't looking to start a new one. I knew, however, I needed to get out of my hibernating behavior and go and have some fun. I really liked to dance. I checked the newspaper for where some singles dances were being held. I also checked the movie schedule to see where a good film was playing in case the dance scene was a drag.

After I arrived and paid my entrance fee I sought out a table with some friendly looking people. The music was good and I was enjoying watching the dancers and their different styles of expression. Now this happened to be the 10th day of the 10th month, October. I kid you not when I tell you that at 10 p.m., Joe sat down next to me and easily started up an interesting conversation. I was enjoying him but in the back of my mind I was asking, "But can he dance?" It was as if he had heard my thoughts when he stood up and led me to the dance floor. We danced until the last song at 1 a.m.

Then Joe and I finished the evening with Irish coffee at a nearby restaurant. I really enjoyed myself for the first time in many months.

It just got better and better and a year and a half later we bought our home. We expected it was where we would live, laugh, love and grow old together. For the most part, we did this. Then our next life chapter of lung cancer came up and bit us both hard. We never expected such a major flip in events would have us living in another state and, for that matter, even continuing to live.

Joe and I returned to Virginia and I believe it was two weeks later that he was told he had been accepted into the program. The seemingly impossible had now become possible.

Okay, the first major hurdle was accomplished. On to the next one. We were told we would have to relocate to North Carolina even if it was on a temporary basis. Joe had to be available within 15 minutes from the hospital for the time period needed when the new lungs, in their fragile state, became available. He also had to be available for the one-year follow-up recovery program after the transplant and in case there was a rejection of the new lungs. That meant that to fill these requirements we would have to find a place to rent near the hospital.

To undergo the strenuous operation, Joe was required to attend daily physical conditioning rehab classes lasting three hours to build up his body. A designated Duke facility was about three miles from the hospital that carried out this program.

As we knew nothing about the area we had to learn what rush hour traffic patterns were like and figure out how the geographic demographics would work for us. We did not know what hour of the day the call might come. We had to find the shortest routes to the hospital to avoid any chance of being too late.

There were financial concerns, too. We were going to have to pay a monthly rental fee along with our house mortgage in Virginia. This would definitely put a strain on the budget. No one tells you how expensive it is to get a lung transplant, even if you have health insurance. It looked like we were going to have to sell our home and make this major move.

Of course, we had no choice. Joe's life was hanging in the balance. Priority one was getting him started in the program. He had to begin it in January, so we had three months to find a place to live in an unfamiliar area and a move to organize. There were so many decisions looming over the whole scenario. I began to feel overwhelmed before I had even packed a box.

"All great changes are preceded by chaos."
~ Deepak Chopra

What I learned:

The English have a great word for how I was feeling. I had been "gobsmacked!" I was being faced once again in my life with the experience of a major loss I did not see coming. I knew that the only way I was going to get through this was by the grace of God. Journaling, meditation, prayer and long-term friendships were really helpful.

Exercise:

Below, I share with you a decision-making tool that can be helpful with the many challenges you might have as you proceed down your path. It is called the Cartesian Coordinates.

List all the things that could happen if you *did* do this.

List all the things that could happen if you *did not* do this.

List all the things that could *not* happen if you *did* do this.

List all the things that could *not* happen if you *did not* do this.

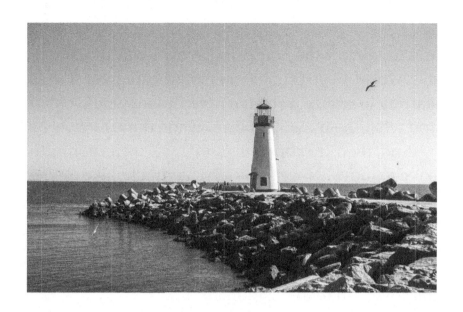

CHAPTER 2:

How Did I Get This Job?

This Wasn't on My Resume

"Most of us can read the writing on the wall; we just assume it's addressed to someone else."
~Ivern Ball

BOY, WAS I EVER feeling challenged. I was already "caregiving" at home because of Joe's condition. At the same time, I had to take care of myself. I was maintaining, in the best ways I could, the daily tasks and upkeep of the house, too. Now I was thrust into this world of a primary personal caregiver. I was starting to realize just what a transplant would entail and what the transplant team wanted me to give.

And then, to top things off, we were going to have to move. Now I was also having to take on the role of organizing the move. I felt like I was way out of my league. I had so much to do my mind was in a constant whirl of questions and tasks. Sometimes I would go up to my room and crawl under the covers in fetal position.

What had happened to my life? It seemed like just a few months ago I was enjoying my work as a psychologist, coach and consultant. Now I was in this new world. What was I doing? Could I really be an asset to Joe in this transplant process? Was this the role for me? I felt like a round peg trying to stuff herself into a square hole.

Due to his increasing debilitation, Joe had become confined to the lower level of our 3200-square-foot house. Stair climbing was daunting to him. To take a bath upstairs it took him 30 minutes to get up the stairs and down the hall to the bathroom with the tub. All other times, he bathed in the sink in the half-bath on the lower level.

Before Joe's symptoms became worse, we used to share chores equally. He would do his laundry and help me fold mine. We would bathe our large dog, Mystique, together. He could scrub her down better than I could. We always enjoyed commissary shopping together and he could carry in the bags. We shared the extensive yardwork with raking, seeding, planting, watering, and tree pruning. He would kill the occasional snakes and voles.

Joe was good at outdoor maintenance like deck, porch, pool, fence, walkways and driveway. I did most of the indoor stuff. At Christmas he would trim the house with Christmas lights while I trimmed the tree. We loved taking our dog on long walks together, including to the beach. We also rode our bikes on beautiful days with our friends. There was a balance and a rhythm to the way we lived together.

As he could do less and less he became increasingly frustrated as he watched more and more being laid on my shoulders. I was trying to maintain the outdoor chores, pool maintenance, washing, cooking, cleaning, dog walking, shopping, etc. These were all, for me, extremely physical activities, and, as I was still in recovery mode myself, I was getting run down.

You see, two years before, I spent five months in the hospital due to several heart surgeries that had me in a fragile state with my heart functioning at only 20% capacity. I lucked out with the insertion of a pacemaker.

The next year I was hospitalized for two more months following an emergency appendectomy that was botched and went septic. A couple of years prior to this I also had emergency surgery on a hernia that had gone septic. I mention these because I've had a few near misses in abrupt endings to my life. Evidently God decided to keep me around. Maybe it was to be Joe's primary personal caregiver and to write this book for you to read. Both serve the purpose and intention for helping others with their own life or death experiences.

With my own hospitalizations I found that, like many patients facing recovery from a serious illness or condition, there were plenty of lonely and scary times in the hospital. I had never been away from home so long. Five days, maybe, but five months? Besides Joe and our neighborhood friends, I really missed my sweet dog, Mystique.

Once in a while, my Joe came to visit me. His daughter would help to get him to whichever hospital or rehab center I was in. Those trips were painful for him. Getting in and out of a vehicle as well as a wheelchair while trying to take in oxygen from his tank involved a lot of exertion with his lungs.

At one time during the appendectomy mess, I was screaming so much with pain I banned all visitors to my room, including Joe. I didn't want him to see me in so much agony as I knew he would be even more stressed emotionally to witness it. I did not want to add to the stress I knew he was already in just getting to the hospital. Unfortunately, my choice to do this only upset him even more.

All of this manifested in a few deep times of depression. I never made it all the way down to despair, but sadness permeated me. I had come close to literally dying of a broken heart. I knew it still held a lot of emotional scarring. When you are lying in a hospital bed for long periods you think too much. Memories with regrets of the past and fears of the future visit you regularly. It is a good sign of recovery when you are beginning to enjoy the present more and more.

One person that helped me with this was my close friend, June. She was a precious gift to me when I was hospitalized the second time. Every night after a long day at work she would drive out of her way to visit me. She ran many errands and just helped brighten my day.

I have written here about some of my personal medical challenges because they gave me experiential knowledge that would help me in my future role of caregiving. Of course then I saw things from a different perspective. We never really know why we have to go through something at the time, do we? The lessons are all about the dos and don'ts and what is helpful and what is not, at least for you.

"When it is dark enough, you can see the stars."
~Ralph Waldo Emerson

When I finally returned home it was an adjustment for us both. Joe had developed his own routines and ways of eating, bathing, cleaning, shopping, getting bills paid and so forth. I was weak and unable to help much for a while. Physical therapy was a godsend to get me back and functioning as a partner again.

Our new normal was not easy to like. With all the separation, we had to get used to living together again with our new physical realities. We both suffered bouts of depression due to our medications and physical states. Joe's depression remained more constant while I tried to be more optimistic. The difference was that my body was trying to recover while his was deteriorating.

There were additional hospital stays for Joe with his collapsed lungs and gall stones removals. Life was incredibly bleak. I would often look in the mirror and ask, "Who are you and what the hell happened to you?" My theme song became "Is This All There Is?"

We were not enjoying each other and with no bright spot for the future showing up, my thoughts were dimmed by remembering so many past struggles, too. I was definitely not living in the joy of the present moment.

Chapter 2: How Did I Get This Job?

> *"We can destroy ourselves by cynicism and disillusion, just as effectively as by bombs."*
> *~Kenneth Clark*

Due to his medical condition, Joe had been forced to retire three years before he had planned to. Therefore, our financial situation had also changed. And now we needed more paid help around the house.

With me no longer physically able to do all the home maintenance, we had to make some adjustments. We closed up the pool. We hired a lawn service company. Therapeutic gardening became too much of a chore and went by the wayside. Dust collected on furniture. The vacuum cleaner felt heavy and hard to push. I could only clean one floor out of three stories at a time. I would do this on alternate weeks. Eventually we had to hire someone to do the heavy cleaning.

The fun pool parties, dinner get-togethers and holiday gatherings were no longer a part of our lives. Interacting with other people, even his grandchildren, was such an exertion for Joe that he'd be worn out within an hour.

We didn't go many places together anymore. It was always a real hassle. Rollators (walkers with wheels) and wheelchairs, oxygen tanks and oxygen concentrators became permanent fixtures. Though useful, they weren't all that easy to manage when leaving home. I had to hoist them up into the back of his car and I also kept a cane handy for me in both of our cars. Going out together became less frequent. As a couple about all we did was watch TV together at night. We grew increasingly isolated.

Joe's depression manifested with him becoming a real curmudgeon and not pleasant to be around. His perceptions of the world were filled with negativity. Talking constantly about how all politicians were terrible was a regular theme. It got pretty boring. He immersed himself in TV. He looked for the flaws in everything and continuously pointed them out. I was pretty sure he was doing the same with his perceptions of me. At least this was how I felt.

As Joe's physical situation declined so did our relationship. There were no more acts of affection unless I gave them. Anniversaries, birthdays, and holidays were left for the most part unacknowledged. To him they were simply one more day to try and get through. This bred a lot of resentment in me. I was not getting the attention or loving energy and appreciation that I needed. The one-sidedness took its toll. I stopped giving the anniversary and birthday gifts and cards. I would still get one Christmas gift for him to put under the tree even though I had none from him. Celebration of anything had become muted.

Joe could handle a lot of ordering or "customer

service" calls by phone but would usually become frustrated with slow and inefficient assistance. He became the stereotype for the "irate customer." Without cussing he could still berate the representatives for their incompetence.

Here was a man who once held top leadership positions on U.S. Naval ships, now reduced to constant re-explanations with incompetent employees. He was definitely not a happy camper and I had to listen to his "piss and vinegar" diatribes. As his disease got worse so did his behavior towards me and others.

I think we both had many moments of complete dislike for one another. Joe's negativity in discussing others got old for me. His own self-esteem was low. The group work and classes the transplant team would later provide in the program did help us see how common this was within an environment such as ours.

Medications, fear, resentment and anger can damage a lot of relationships. Professionally I know this. But when you are in the midst of it every day for over two or three years, patience with the behavior runs thin. There is a saying that if you put a "normal" person in a room often enough with a neurotic one, you will end up with two neurotics. I could see that this was happening to me.

(I want to note here that within six months after

his surgery, Joe began to really turn this around and our mutually loving acts returned once more. More about this later.)

To get some space from this I spent a lot of time upstairs and on the computer in my office trying to keep up with my ongoing coaching classes and clients. I connected with many online groups as well as spiritually uplifting people across the country. It helped bring in a few rays of sunshine to the dark cloud that hung over our home.

Though I couldn't leave him alone for long, I would try and get out occasionally to socialize a little. Some days just meandering around a mall for an hour would feel therapeutic as well as a walk with Mystique.

I did always look forward to lunch dates with different friends. Listening to what was going on in other people's lives helped to take me out of my own dark version of mine for a little while. Often one finds, though, that you really would not want to trade places with them, and they may be thinking the same about you.

I also got together with my friend, June. We would meet for lunch and a movie about three times a month. During our "chick dates," I would try not to complain. She knew how difficult things were at home anyway. As we are both psychologists we knew how to tweak each other's buttons in healthy ways. We would usually end up belly-laughing and get the great endorphins flowing. There were other benefits — I would lighten up to a better mood and when I returned home I would be more pleasant to Joe. I could talk with him about the movie or some funny things that June and I had shared. Dinner seemed to taste better and the air felt lighter.

"A good friend is cheaper than therapy."
~Author Unknown

What I learned:

Isolation is a killer. When nobody is helping to boost you up, you end up flat on your face. Support groups of like-minded people, even on the Internet, can help you change perspective. Keeping your mind active with upbeat interests and ongoing communication is therapeutic.

Exercise:

This little exercise can help to lighten you up:

Stand in front of your mirror, look deep into your eyes and say the words, "Woe is me." Say it again emphasizing a different word. "Woe is ME." Again, "Woe IS me." Again, "WOE is me." Do it about 3 times. See how you feel a little differently each time. You may just start giggling. ("You can also do this with "I am a loser.")

Now go through the process with a smile on your

face but change the word Woe to Wow. "WOW is me." Again, "Wow is ME." Again, "Wow IS me." Notice that you also experience different feelings here, too. Which do you prefer? You are in charge. Just keep saying it with the preferred inflection throughout your day. Also remember that how you look to yourself in the mirror is how you look to others as you share your preferences.

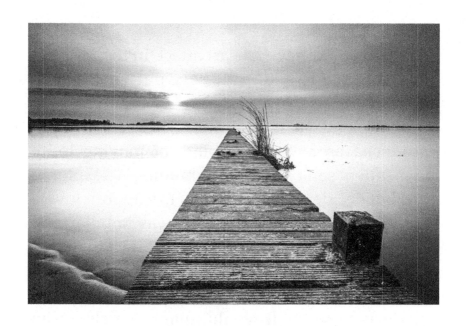

CHAPTER 3:

Where Am I Going and How Do I Get There?

The Maze of Mania

"If you're going through hell, keep going."
~ Winston Churchill

THE THREE MONTHS BETWEEN mid-September and the first part of December were full of confusion, anger, fear, frustration and incredible overwhelm.

I feared I would have a heart attack in the midst of it all. Now that would really have put a damper on Joe getting his transplant.

A couple of years before, our financial advisor introduced us to the possibility of moving to an independent senior living community. We explored a few but decided we didn't want to leave our lovely home for several more years. It was familiar and comfortable and making that big of a change was not all that attractive to us at that time. Two years later, the whole idea would become a lifesaver for what was to come. It would, unfortunately, mean leaving our home much sooner than expected and putting it on the market. More about that later.

We knew of several places in Virginia that were of interest, but we knew nothing of avenues in North Carolina. I contacted a state senior services advocate and told her of our situation. On our next visit to Durham one of the independent senior living centers invited us to stay with them for a free weekend to see what it would be like to live at their community. This was a great marketing ploy. The people were quite pleasant, but the location was extremely unacceptable. There were too many hilly areas that endangered my maneuverability of Joe's wheelchair outside between buildings. Walking our big dog, Mystique, twice a day would also have put me into real danger for major falls. I just had to stay intact for the care of both Joe and our sweet pet.

Chapter 3: Where Am I Going and How Do I Get There?

I have been a pretty adaptable trooper most of my life. As a former military wife, I had moved 13 times over a 20-year period. However, I had not had to do that for the past 18 years. I was coming from a lovely place that had 3200 square feet. Now I was being shown spaces not much larger than my garage. The very loud question in my mind was, "You want me to what?"

I stood in the so-called living room of one place and started to cry. The reality of the complete loss of my former life swooped in and I began to grieve. Everything in me was shouting, "No! Please God, No!" I almost collapsed as I tried as hard as I could to fit my square self into a round hole.

> *"When you come to the end of your rope,*
> *tie a knot and hang on."*
> *~ Franklin D. Roosevelt*

We also found that many places that said they were pet friendly really meant if your pet weighed less than 40 lbs., they were friendly. Our wonderful fur baby weighed 80 lbs. That diminished our list of what was available to us in a considerable way.

We finally went to a rather upscale place just to look around. It was in the area of the last one we visited. As soon as we walked in, our vibes changed. As we were led on a tour with a lovely lady, Joe and I were feeling more and more comfortable. The place had a wonderful ambience to it with which we both connected.

In our meeting with both the Executive and Sales Directors we explained fully what our situation was with the short timetable, the size of our dog and how she was a necessary therapeutic assist for both of us. She had been with us since we rescued her 16 years before. We weren't about to cast her off now. We also explained that we had recently decided to put our home on the housing market so we could afford this new way of life.

There are many nice amenities incorporated into the rental cost for these centers. This one included housekeeping, landscaping, maintenance of everything, and two daily-prepared meals. There were real chefs as opposed to short-order cooks preparing your food. You could eat in their formal dining room or have some of your meals delivered to you. Not having to think about making meals was a great appeal to me then.

They had a great exercise room with good machines for you to use at any time of the day. Daily instructor-led exercise classes were also available. There were many activities, outings, trips, etc. The whole set-up was like living in a nice hotel with ongoing room, concierge and shuttle service.

The location was 15 minutes from Duke Hospital and the lovely surroundings outside were flat. I could handle the wheelchair and dog walks easily.

However, they only had one option of availability that had just become open that week. Would we like to see it?

It was in one of the 20 cottages that was separate from the main building. I quickly agreed as I had noticed them when we entered the area. Joe begged off as his energy was spent. It was easier to not have to wheel him over there as my own energy was low. I brought his chair in and out of the car and wheeled him around buildings several times already that day.

The director called the people living there to get their permission to bring me over. Due to some family situation, they were having to vacate by the end of November...the day after my birthday. It perfectly fit our timetable.

When I walked in I was thrilled by all the light coming in from all of the windows. The decor was a nice pale yellow and white, which was similar to our home in Virginia. There was a fenced-in patio that our dog and my flower pots could enjoy and the space was 1500 square feet plus a garage. I liked it a lot.

I did a quick chat with the present residents and found out they used to live in the same town we were coming from in Virginia and knew our neighborhood well. Now the community is made up of 100 senior men and women from all across the country, Canada, Europe and South America. What were the chances I would run into these people from our hometown who were vacating that space at that particular time? Talk about a sign...a feather could have floated down in front of me and knocked me over.

"Coincidence is God's way of remaining anonymous."
~Albert Einstein

Going back to the sales office, I could see Joe didn't want to stay much longer but he could tell I had been revived with what I had just encountered. We still had the issues with the resident cost and size of our dog. When the two women heard about the conversation I had with the residents they looked at each other with a knowing smile. It seemed they were sensing something as well. Perhaps a solution could be found. It seemed like a bit of divine confirmation was at play.

We left with a sample contract, floor plans and the kindness of the directors. They knew we were in a life and death situation and they were both lovers of any size dogs. They said they would keep in touch with us. However, we didn't know if we would ever see them again.

We returned home still not knowing where our next address was going to be. On our first trip to Durham we had stayed at a hotel that would accommodate the handicapped and allowed for dogs. With a couple of breakfasts there, it had cost us $1000 for the 4 nights and 5 days. The rates were discounted for people in the Duke Hospital transplant programs. It looked like we were going to have to come up with another $1000 for the next trip down to Durham. Doing this again to buy us (literally) some time until we could find a place seemed like our only option. At least I knew the North Carolina Senior Center Alliance would be helping us in our search.

Now we had to get ourselves ready for a huge move to who knew where. Even though it was for Joe to get another chance at life, the task ahead was "looming large." This was truly a huge reality bite in the butt. Organization for a move was not my forte. I couldn't even pack suitcases efficiently.

With so much upkeep involved, it wasn't likely that we would live in a home of this size again. After almost 20 years of accumulation of "stuff," much would have to be eliminated before we moved. The realization was there that I would be doing all of the legwork.

Exhaustion plagued me. I was scared, frustrated, angry and sad over this huge change that was now being thrust upon us. Guilt for having these feelings would wash over me. We were being given an unbelievable opportunity for Joe to have a second chance at life. Yet there was so much "letting go" of the familiar. It was daunting. There were no guarantees either of a happy ending.

That really didn't help our situation one bit. My

kicking and screaming resistance over this sudden change kept the stress level high. Luckily, God had allowed me my tantrums before and still helped me to feel loving arms around me. This came with meditation, visits with friends, phone calls from out of the blue from old friends, and just being lovingly touched by Nature on my walks, drives and even the movies.

> *"I know God will not give me anything*
> *I can't handle. I just wish that*
> *He didn't trust me so much."*
> *~Mother Teresa*

I had heard about estate sales and how they could provide an efficient way to dispose of household property. I decided to look into those. I contacted three companies and had them come over and explain to us how they worked. How could they really be of use to us in our present situation?

One of them was an auctioneer and said he could take our whole house and auction everything off. Of course, we had no idea how much the house would sell for at an auction. He would be pricing everything. He did a lot of farm houses and ranches out west. I could imagine him auctioning cattle and horses as well. This "good old boy" just didn't feel like a fit for us and so we tried another person.

A well-dressed gentleman arrived the next day. He said he would be the realtor for the house sale but would subcontract out to another company to sell our personal property. He was professional and business like but somehow didn't feel quite right for the job either. There was no sense of "connection" with him. Our home and goods were just business commodities.

Finally, two women came by to give us their pitch. They went off throughout the house looking at our property in an appreciative manner. I began to feel a connection with them. They had performed many estate sales throughout Virginia and had pictures that showed the sales on their website. It definitely had the woman's touch. They were able to express their understanding of what it was like to let go of so many pieces associated with fond memories. China, crystal, silver, artwork, furniture, clothing, tools, holiday furnishings, yard-work machinery, gardening supplies, and pool accessories were all among what had to go.

They gave us a reality bite about price expectations. For instance, we might prize all of our sterling silver pieces we received as wedding gifts but they did not hold the same value for the market today. The demand for them was no longer as great as it had been back in our day. We had to accept that we would never get the value of what our possessions were truly worth to us. Each woman had been through major changes later in life herself and could appreciate a lot of our concerns.

Another sign for me was that they used both a Catholic youth charity and a women's shelter for everything we wanted donated. I, too, had made numerous donations to these groups in the past. My task was going to be to sort through everything to separate items meant for moving and others for the estate sale. They would take care of all the cleaning, polishing, tagging and pricing.

One woman's husband was a real estate agent. She also had a contracting business we could use for repairs in getting the house ready for market. They were almost like a one-stop shop. The house would be staged with the sale items over a long weekend. People could be looking at the house as well as shopping through the items for sale. Anything left would be donated, tossed or moved into the sale of another estate for possible future sales.

Antique owners and silversmiths would also be contacted to give them advanced notice of the sale. It would be advertised on the internet and posters would be put up all over the area. We had to trust them and let them do what they were best at by getting out of their way. There was a strong sense they were good, honest people who were truly interested in easing our situation in all ways that they could.

We arranged for the sale to take place in January. We would have to be in North Carolina by that time but all would be in their care, so we could make the move. Overwhelm began to subside and I finally began to breathe again.

I contacted a moving company and set a date to get us and our left-over worldly goods to North Carolina by the end of the year. We still had no address. As we were being financially challenged in every way, I tried to take some shortcuts by doing everything I could by myself with sorting and some packing.

> *I often think I can't do this anymore but then I realize what choice do I have?"*
> *~Justin Blaney*

I had a three-story house to sort through. I also had shopping, cooking, washing, cleaning, dog walking, and medical appointments to keep. I bought boxes at Home Depot in addition to the ones the movers brought over. I thought I could manage this given I had a month. I had managed a couple of small, quick moves to apartments when I was younger and single. This move was nothing like that.

Eighteen years of accumulation in 3200 square feet and a large yard with a pool entailed sorting through tools, supplies, kitchenware, clothing, and files. There were boxes in the attic, pantry items, home décor, electronics, office materials and a lot of furniture both indoors and outdoors. When one thinks they will be living in a place forever, there isn't a pressing need to reduce the accumulation in such great amounts.

Through the years we had made many donations and had yard sales. Our home never looked cluttered and was tastefully decorated. But by the time I started going through everything I found a lot more "stuff" than was needed behind cabinet and closet doors and furniture drawers. If it had all been on the outside I think we could have starred on the Hoarders show. I had to admit that I was a saver. A lot of what we had was either for sentimental value or for "I might need this for something else." It all reflected both the past and the future. It wasn't really needed in the present.

It often felt like a part of me was disappearing with the boxes I packed or marked for donations. Letting go of everything became my biggest lesson for this time of my life. I even moved the "Let It Go" song from the movie *Frozen* onto my favorite playlist. Besides this I added more walks with Mystique, drives through the park and even some better food choices. I knew that keeping my energy up would be absolutely necessary.

What I learned:

Letting go meant letting go. Resistance was my tether that kept me from moving forward into freedom. Fear and Hope often tie together. We hope our fears will not become realized. It is good to remember that fear is mostly:

F***k Everything And Run.
or
Face Everything And Rise

Exercises:

Exercise #1. That's it…exercise! This is both for your body and your mind. Whatever you focus on can either drain you of energy or increase it. Obviously, fear can flush your energy right down the tubes.

Since I am more of an outdoors person, walking and bike riding have been my exercise of choice. Swimming had also been handy with a pool in the back yard. That is until we had to close it up. I get spontaneous urges, which is why I chose these modes for myself. Getting dressed to drive to a gym and workout with weights did not hold my interest for too many months. Besides, I know I am undisciplined when it comes to exercise.

Exercise #2. Be aware of what foods you consume and of any urges to eat away your emotions and overwhelm. I found that eating crunchy things like baby carrots, celery sticks and even a few thin crackers with a dip of hummus satisfied me most times. I did have my binges on ice cream or cookies but not often. I could tell the zap of energy they took on my body the next day. Don't make excuses for those binges like, "I've had a tough day and I deserve it." Well, at least not more than once a week.

Exercise #3. Try to get in just 20–30 minutes a day of focusing on something positive or beautiful or humorous. Take a fast-clip walk or run, preferably out in Nature listening to upbeat music. Read some beautiful poetry. Listen to guided imagery or soothing meditation tapes. Trade sugary "comfort foods" which cause real "downer moods" for tasty, lighter fare. Watch funny movies. Share funny animal videos with online buddies. You know best what really picks you up. As Nike says, "Just do it!"

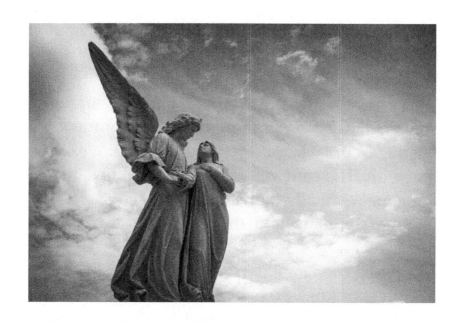

CHAPTER 4:

Is This the Yellow Brick Road?

Where Are the Munchkins?

"The future rewards those who press on. I don't have time to feel sorry for myself. I don't have time to complain. I'm going to press on."
~Barack Obama

Almost three weeks after our house hunting trip to Durham we received a letter from our favorite independent senior living center. After talking with their corporate office, permission had been given to allow us to rent the lovely cottage I had toured. Due to the life and death situation Joe was in, some waivers had been put in place which included our big dog. A price had been negotiated that we could live with. The contract was signed and faxed back to them. We finally had an address! I contacted the moving company and the date was set. We had three weeks.

Having been a military wife with over 13 moves in 20 years, I knew some of what was needed. However, all household moves had been paid for and arranged by the United States Army. My former husband and I only oversaw the packing of the boxes.

Our toughest move came when he was assigned overseas. We could only take a certain weight allowance of our goods and the rest had to be packed up and put in storage. As usual, the contracted company did all of this while we did the sorting. At least we knew when we returned stateside after three years that we would have access to our stored possessions again.

With the move to North Carolina with Joe, whatever we left would be gone for good. Although storage areas were available, they were costly. We were already on thin ice with both the rental cost and the mortgage hanging over us. Besides, we had already come to terms with that when we chose to have the company for the estate sale take over that hassle.

Chapter 4: Is This the Yellow Brick Road?

I ordered bulk supplies of packing boxes and materials to supplement those from the movers. These I got from the internet. A bulk package of a variety of box sizes was cheaper than buying them separately. I found I could do better on buying the expensive wardrobe boxes separately at Home Depot. I learned I would save myself some frustration if I also bought several dispensers to more quickly tape the boxes without trying to find the darn end of the tape roll every time I picked it up.

We asked Joe's son and daughter to come over before I started packing to take whatever they wanted. Their choices filled a pickup truck and car but only made a small dent in what was left. It was an emotionally difficult task for them as they watched their father have to leave his home. Instead of a 30-minute drive from their respective homes, they would now be many hours away.

About two years prior to our move Joe had to stop creating his beautiful remote-control model airplanes. Now these were not just your balsa wood pieces you would put together at the kitchen table. These planes were flown at real airfields. The designs had fuselages of around six feet with wingspans of five to seven feet. Our garage was devoted to the hobby.

As a perfectionist craftsman, Joe turned them into real works of art. The amount of detail that went into them took many hours of labor. Each one was a real "big boy's toy." The parts and engines were pretty expensive. Yet it is all relative. Skiing, sailing and golfing are expensive pastimes as well. At least I knew where he was spending most of the time...in the garage. The sad part was how Joe's depression increased when he could no longer work on his beautiful creations.

Out of the blue came my angel. Peg has been a great friend for over 30 years. Indeed, ours is one of the best friendships I have ever had. We have shared many ongoing-life experiences with great support for one another. We had both experienced divorce. As I was re-entering the dating scene she was very helpful. As we had both been former military wives, we still were members of the same-faith military family communities. We were not divorced from them.

However, we did join groups for the divorced, separated and widowed (DSW) as well. We discovered other women and some men who were like-minded with strong spiritual roots. Members of these groups had experienced the traumatic loss of loved ones and relationships. Through the sharing of other people's stories with acceptance and non-judgment, close connections often evolved.

Of course we also learned which characters were just using these groups to meet people for one-night stands. Peg was one of my several friends who would give me a heads-up on who some of these were. We all watched out for each other. At least five of us would spend many weekends both screaming with laughter and sobbing with disappointment over the whole dating endeavors we all encountered. Besides the healthy male relationships I have had, I will always treasure my women friends.

In time, Peg met and fell in love with a wonderful man. Although she quit going with our group to singles dances and the DSW groups, we still stayed in close contact. I was privileged to be at her wedding to Bob. He became another dear friend to me.

Eventually Joe came into the picture and both Peg and Bob, after sizing him up, welcomed him into the fold. We spent many holidays together even though Joe and I lived about three hours away. Luckily for us Peg had several family members in the area of Virginia I had moved to. It was there that I had met Joe. We were often included in their family gatherings.

We had kept close as the various medical situations arose for all of us. However, we didn't travel back and forth as much anymore. The three-hour trip between Virginia Beach and the Washington DC area had become four hours. A lot of construction and bumper-to-bumper lane clogs brought on a lot of frustration. We also had our big dog and putting her in a kennel was costly.

After hearing all about what was going on with our new adventure, Peg picked up the stress in my voice about handling the move. She immediately offered to come to our house in Virginia for a weekend before our move and help me with the packing. She would come with her husband, whom Joe had always enjoyed. The two men could not physically help, Bob had a heart condition, but they could entertain each other. She had a lot of experience with the task and was a master at organization. This was no small offer of service to Joe and me. The gratitude in my heart for her and Bob was and is still overflowing.

"Friends are kisses blown to us by angels."
-Author Unknown

What we accomplished in that weekend I could not have done on my own over several weeks. I needed her expertise and energy to become efficient and effective myself with this tall task. With her help, items were sorted quickly by size for different boxes. It was uncanny to me how she knew how to place items just so in a box to save space. She used plastic wrap, newspapers, articles of clothing, bedding and even Mystique's stuffed animals to safely wrap the items.

Her labeling of the boxes with contents and the rooms they served saved me hours of unpacking on the other end. She thought of things that would be needed right away and made special packages to bring in the cars. In three days we accomplished

Chapter 4: Is This the Yellow Brick Road?

what would have taken me three weeks to do. I know by the time she left, 90% of the job was done. Peg was just about crawling out the door with exhaustion as we said our goodbyes. She had truly given her all.

Since the movers were coming the next day, I continued to work until midnight and fell onto my bare mattress totally exhausted. The movers showed up around 9 a.m. They finished the packing of whatever was left and even called in two more packers to help. If I had known they would do this, I may have gotten another couple of hours of sleep.

I had put everything that was not to go with us into one large room. They were not to touch those boxes as they had been designated for the estate sale. Unfortunately, I now believe one important box had mistakenly been moved into that room as well.

I had to direct five movers as they picked up boxes and articles to be moved out onto the truck. I had to make sure they got everything while omitting what was to be left for the estate sale. I was moving between the three floors, consisting of three bedrooms, loft, room over the garage, family room, living room, dining room, kitchen, three bathrooms, closets, garage and outdoor deck. I will say that for the most part, they did a good job of following directions. It was not their first rodeo.

The movers left mid-afternoon and headed for our new home. I took about an hour to vacuum up what I could and put the trash cans on the curb. Whatever was left would have to be done by the company running the estate sale. This was part of their service. I packed up both of our cars with suitcases, food, wheel chairs, rollators, oxygen tanks and our dog's food, blanket and her toys.

We said one last goodbye to our home and headed out, each in our own car. As I drove off, I kept saying to myself, "Donna has left the building." I wasn't feeling sad. I think I was feeling more concerned about getting to North Carolina as soon as we could. I simply wanted everything over and done with.

It felt better to finally move my focus from leaving the house to getting to our new place. As an Army wife I had led a nomadic life. In that respect I was just "moving on" once again. I was more interested in getting everything into the new place and not worrying about the particulars until the next day. I had done this with all my prior moves. In my mind, once I am done with something I am done with it. On to the next adventure!

My main concern was Joe driving himself the whole four hours. I would be following him hoping he would be all right and not get too tired. Oxygen tanks had been loaded into his car so his supply was good. If he needed to pull over to rest, I knew he would do so.

Chapter 4: Is This the Yellow Brick Road?

Our dog, Mystique, rode with him. It was important to Joe to have her with him for company. She had more room to lie down in his car as well. However, she would have been a problem for him if he had to get out of his car without help. She could have easily slipped out unleashed.

To help lower my stressful state as I drove my car, I played loud music on my radio and sang along. It felt playful and no one could judge my lack of talent or choice of music.

I was afraid of getting separated from Joe on this long trek and not being there if he needed me. We stopped halfway along the route for bathroom breaks and a short walk for the dog.

All was going well until the last hour of the trip. Joe's car had a GPS system but my older car did not. It had become dark and my yellow brick road of Interstate became unfamiliar two-lane curvy roads. It left me agitated and wondering if he was lost. I sure was.

At last we arrived at our new address without incident. The movers had arrived an hour before and were waiting for us. We had all forgotten to exchange cell-phone numbers with each other. They didn't know where we were or when we would show up.

Fortunately, both of the independent senior living center's directors had stayed late making sure our place was ready with new paint and carpeting upgrades completed. We were welcomed with our key and two full dinners laid in for our arrival. The movers began unloading the truck.

We did not know they were planning to do this. We expected them to unload the next morning. They told us they were already assigned to another move back in Virginia the next day and would be traveling back there that night.

To our amazement they unloaded the truck, put the furniture in place everywhere, set up the beds and stacked boxes neatly along all the walls and the garage. Our bewildered dog seemed to be okay staying outside on our new patio while all this was going on. Joe watched from his wheelchair trying to give direction where he could. This was his first sight of the place.

After about three hours, and it was nearing midnight, everything was inside and the movers left. I fed all three of us. We quietly sat and looked at each other. It was done. We were strangers in a strange land.

I helped Joe get his bi-pap on and his oxygen condenser hooked up in his new room. We were exhausted. I put sheets and blankets on the beds and we crawled in. Joe wanted our dog to lie down next to him, but she was bewildered and didn't want to let me out of her sight either. She didn't know which room to sleep in, so she used the hall

Chapter 4: Is This the Yellow Brick Road?

corridor as her central point to try all the rooms out throughout the night.

As you who are caregivers know, it takes a while to tend to your loved one and make sure they are settled before you can begin to get yourself prepared for rest. I think most would agree that rest is whatever time you can capture between listening for wheezing, uncontrolled coughing, violent hacking, or even the thud of possible falls.

You can be awakened abruptly when there is the sudden call for help because something is threatening their ability to breathe. There might be a kink in the cannula line or the oxygen has suddenly run out. There can be the painful leg cramps and or excruciating pain from a collapsed lung or even gall stones. Like you, I kept the number of the ambulance on speed dial.

"I used to go away for weeks in a state of confusion."
~ Albert Einstein

It took Joe and me about a month to adjust to our new environment. First of all, I now had to walk Mystique twice a day. I was used to just opening up our back door to let her out into a large yard. She no longer had that kind of space or accessibility. Our walks together, however, would be a blessing and necessary for both of us. I'll speak of this again later.

There was plenty more "yellow brick road" to travel down. I did spend a lot of time and many wrong turns learning the whereabouts of the best drug stores, food markets, malls, post office, churches, libraries, gas stations, Urgent Care centers, appliance centers, car inspection stations, mechanics, banks, etc. We also had to get new state driver licenses and registrations along with new voter registration cards.

At our senior center, there were welcomes, orientation meetings, menus to choose from and preferred seating times to select. It was different from just being the two of us eating whatever we could find in our freezer and quick meals I would make on the weekends.

Meals now were "chef prepared" and pretty good. Of course anything is good when someone else is cooking it. Most nights I would wheel Joe over to the main building and the dining room. We would try to sit at different tables to help us to socialize with some of the other residents. The kindness and concern among the people for us and one another was quite genuine. We were really being invited into community living again. It was a good change from the isolated state we had drifted into back in Virginia.

Though we moved into our new space the first week of December, I really could not get into decorating for Christmas. I couldn't set up our 7-foot tree by myself and did not even know for sure if it was going to fit. I also did not know which of the many boxes yet to be unpacked contained the ornaments.

I was used to decorating a house of three stories both inside and outside. Our Virginia home had even won a "best in show" award several years before. This year a couple of poinsettia plants, candles and several of our pretty angel figurines were the best I could muster while playing Christmas music. Every day, however, we were able to enjoy the main building's lovely decorations and festive spirit among the staff and some of the other residents.

Throughout the rest of the month I tried to unpack more of the heavy boxes and get our new home set up. After a while and when our environment felt comfortable, Joe and I felt happy with the choices we had made.

"Every new beginning comes from some other beginning's end."
~ Seneca

What I learned:

Ask for help sooner from those who know how to do the task. A stitch in time saves nine. Remember that the munchkins knew a lot more about the Land of Oz than Dorothy did. But don't be too hard on yourself. If you have never been through a daunting challenge before, you don't know what you don't know. The lessons you learn can now be part of your tool kit for offering help to others when you find them as bewildered as you were.

Exercise:

With enrollment in the Duke Hospital transplant program, we were given a Primary Personal Caregiver Manual and demonstration sheets. There were mandatory classes filled with so much information it was overwhelming. However, they gave us a working knowledge of terminology. These helped us form good questions that could be thoroughly answered in the classes or by any member of the transplant teams. The instructors were readily able to help us move through the huge challenge we were enduring. I learned more about what Joe had been going through than he ever told me... Men! We both learned together what was next in this serious process.

If you are not enrolled in a program, my suggestion to you is to ask your physicians if you can partake of some classes held at your hospital where your loved one is being treated. See if you can obtain written information on the condition of your own loved one that is specifically for primary personal care givers. If they don't have it, ask if it can be obtained from other hospitals.

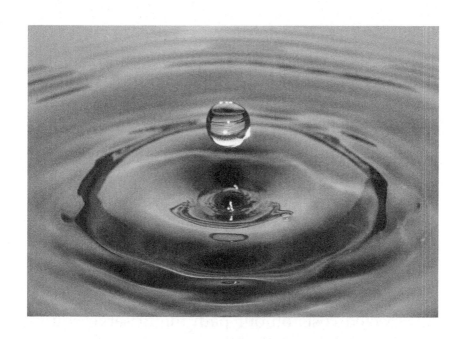

CHAPTER 5:

How Much Did You Say That Would Cost?

You're Kidding, Right?

"I don't like money, actually, but it quiets my nerves."
~Joe Louis

YOU CAN'T GET THROUGH something like this without talking about the financial hurdles that are also present. Getting a transplant involves more than what is covered by insurance. We really had our ups and downs with all the costs. We were between two financial commitment worlds of our home in Virginia and our new one in North Carolina.

I want to share with you the financial changes we encountered that we had never planned for. Perhaps this will be helpful to give you a "heads up" approach to your own situations. Examples of unexpected costs on our path might serve you in not being as blind-sided as we were. We did come through all of them, though, and are still standing.

Through our initial orientation at the independent senior living center, Joe and I learned about cultural area performances, activities and community events for which we could sign up. Though they looked inviting it would take us almost a year to get fully involved. We were still dealing with the costs we were encountering on a daily basis of just moving in and of course the out-of-pocket costs related to Joe's health.

We had to buy a new washer and dryer. The TV, phone and computers needed to be hooked up to new Wi-Fi and cable systems. New program packages were expensive. Joe, thankfully, was knowledgeable in this area and knew what was needed.

He was able to supervise the setups and installations and feel like he was contributing.

Some medical equipment, over-the-counter medications, nutritional and first aid stock-ups not covered by medical insurance had to be purchased. New North Carolina registrations, license plates and personal property fees and taxes were necessary.

This was in addition to still trying to carry a mortgage on our former home with the monthly utilities, association fees, taxes and upkeep. Add to that the steep rent for our new home. At least here the services that were included would free us up from the costs associated with the house. I had a new appreciation for all the headaches the rich probably had with keeping up with everything in their world...Not!

"Money doesn't talk, it swears."
~Bob Dylan, "It's Alright, Ma (I'm Only Bleeding)"

Remember, our former home was up for sale in Virginia. The realtor called several times to get my okay and additional money to upgrade the house. After the estate sale they were focused on getting it even more ready for putting it on the market. Paint, woodwork, landscaping, appliances, cabinetry, and carpet cleaning were needed and cost a lot. I was writing checks adding up to over $25,000. I figured it was temporary, as when the house sold I would be getting it back.

Knowing the circumstances we were in with Joe's transplant process, the Virginia bank officer was allowing us to hold off on the mortgage payments. With the house on the market they knew the bank would be the first to be paid in full once it sold. It was such a relief for us not to have to cover the mortgage.

Two months later, after the house had been fixed up and staged, we received a call from an unknown bank branch credit office in Texas. Joe happened to be in the hospital recovering from a collapsed lung when the phone call came. With great efficiency and brusque manner, a credit manager told him that our former agreement was off the table. The bank officer who had worked this out with Joe was no longer with the bank. Since the agreement was not in writing, it was ruled null and void by the collections department. We never even had a say. We had to immediately pay three months of mortgage along with late-fee penalties. We couldn't. They foreclosed.

In my mind I threw spears of demeaning judgment at the whole banking industry and their underhanded tactics. I wasn't too crazy about the real estate industry either. Both had really let us down.

No home. No money to be made on it. No return of my upgrade monies. There was nothing left for us to even hire an attorney to go up against the whole raft of bank lawyers. It was over. The bridge had been burned and so had we.

I set up a page on the "GoFundMe" site and several dear friends made generous contributions. I wasn't surprised at who did...but really surprised at who did not.

The money we did receive from the fund helped us in paying the ongoing high expense of daily parking fees at the hospital.

"Never idealize others.
They will never live up to your expectations."
~Leo Buscaglia

After a week or two of ranting and tears, we decided to look at how much more money we now had. No mortgage payment. No utilities or association fees. No landscaping or pool costs. No more property taxes. We could now handle the monthly rent and have a little left over. What really hurt us was not having the $70,000 to $90,000 net profit we thought we would get on the house sale. With our fixed incomes, it would have helped tremendously over the next three or four years.

Strangely enough, it felt as though we could now focus on our real priority, Joe's transplant. Our present needs were being taken care of with what we had. We could see that everything in the last four months had been provided and laid out before us. Why shouldn't this situation be positive as well? This would become a theme for us.

One thing I would definitely suggest that you do early in your pre-transplant program is to work both with your mortgage company and the financial advisors on your transplant team. There may be some kind of programs with loans of which most of us are simply unaware. Not knowing ahead of time what was going to happen to us, we did not check into this. We thought we would be ok. Live and learn…again and again.

> *"And we know that all things work together for good to those who love God."*
> *~ Romans 8:28*

What I learned:

Other people are living their own lives. We have no idea about why they make the choices they do. Often, though, they provide a mirror for us to see how making those same choices ourselves can affect others in ways that probably weren't intended. Their business is none of mine. My life is my business alone. My choices are my choices alone.

However, I am never alone. My faith has shown me that God, Source or Creator is all about my own business. I am always receiving guidance (when I listen) to making better choices. I often find that these choices result in less fear, more confidence and lightness of being.

Exercise:

Make a list of everyone for whom you feel resentment. This can be singular (your cousin Vinnie) or include whole groups of people (all of your in-laws). You may even add industries (the healthcare policymakers). There is always the government to add to your list. When you have put everybody you can think of on that list, take 10 deep breaths. Go to each name or group and in writing tell them exactly why you resent them.

When you finish and feel you have gotten the resentments and anger out of your system, or at least decreased the intensity, take 10 more deep breaths. Now, in your continuing meditation, go back to each one and ask why they might resent you resenting them. Listen quietly with no comments. Write down what you hear and feel. Surprising revelations may heal some of that pain.

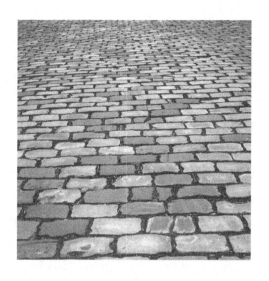

CHAPTER 6:

Where Do We Go Now for This Transplant?

The Bricks Are Pretty Dusty

*"We know what we are,
but know not what we may be."
~ William Shakespeare*

THE PREPARATION PROGRAM FOR Joe's transplant surgery was quite intensive. No one knew how long this would be. Joe and I are independent types of people. His now total dependence on me went against the grain for both of us. We had to accept that this was just a way of life.

Part of my caregiver responsibilities was being present or within close proximity for all of his pre-op requirements. Most mornings were spent at the Cardiac and Pulmonary rehab facility. Joe had to go through strenuous progressive exercise conditioning. His body had to be brought up to a certain level of strength to give him the best chance of success at surviving the highly delicate transplant operation. This took three hours five times a week.

On top of all the daily conditioning, Joe had some other painful experiences to contend with. One night he awoke with very labored breathing. His symptoms mirrored that of a collapsed lung, which he had experienced several months before. This resulted in another ambulance ride to the hospital and a few days of recovery.

His transplant team quickly scheduled him back into his exercise program at rehab. The same thing happened when he had to have some terribly painful gall stones removed. The team had him back into his extensive exercise regimen almost immediately upon release from the hospital.

This seemed counterintuitive to me. I thought an extended period of rest would be needed. Not according to his transplant team. They knew what they were doing. They also, not so subtly, let me

Chapter 6: Where Do We Go Now for This Transplant?

know that too. This was not my area of expertise — it was theirs.

There was no quiet waiting room at the rehab facility. There was continuous traffic up and down the small hall you could sit in. The noise from machines and instructors working with the patients was a constant din. I knew I couldn't last three hours in that environment. I chose a variety of ways to spend my time.

It was too far from home for another roundtrip to the facility. As it was closer, I would drive to the city library sometimes and wander among the books and magazines. Other days, I would visit a small mall and window shop. Sometimes I would sit in my car in the parking lot and call friends and relatives around the country. Other days, I would read, or play games on my iPad. That went on for six months.

Two or three times a week we had to go to Duke University Hospital. There were lab tests to be run and continuous appointments with surgeons, a nutritionist, social worker and psychiatrist. We would have to fit in lunch between visits with them. We would head to the hospital food court. Our dining companions were about a hundred other people. The food wasn't bad. There was a lot of variety to include chain eateries and the prices were a little better than outside.

A big part of the program involved mandatory attendance at three-hour classes and lectures at the hospital. The ones given at the rehab center lasted about two hours. Huge amounts of information were crammed into that time and our brains. We had to learn everything that we definitely had to do, as well as everything that we maybe would have to do, before, during and after the transplant surgery. Once it was "go time" there wouldn't be time to learn — we had to move into action.

Bi-monthly sessions involved gatherings with a good social worker. She helped address some of the concerns of the primary personal caregivers. The groups did not include the patient so there could be more openness in sharing those concerns. The sociologist who led the groups had been part of the transplant teams for several years. I was definitely helped by her experience. It was good for me to have a professional colleague available to play the role I played in my business life, that of professional listener.

With her help I could deal with the issues of negative talk and disappointment in relationship expectations. I was reminded of how my own disappointment in myself and feelings of ineptness were adding to my distress.

We went over a lot of techniques and strategies I used with my former clients and selected which ones would be helpful to me in my present situation. Some of these I have been sharing with you at the end of the chapters. Wearing unfamiliar shoes can sometimes make someone forget the knowledge they already have inside them.

Several other classes were led by a psychologist. These were for both the transplant patient and the primary personal caregiver. Coping skills around medical side effects, depression, mood swings, and good de-stressing techniques were offered. It was a thorough program given over several weeks. I had taught some classes on stress reduction years ago at a university. I could appreciate the strengths of the information in what was a new arena for me.

All of these classes held a wide variety of families. They were doing their best to assist their loved one on their path of freedom from their awful pain and darkness in which they tried to survive. They came from all over the United States and several other countries. We saw people who wore raggedy clothes to others with expensive labels. Many spoke with country slang and others articulated from higher levels of education.

Some situations were beyond what most of us can imagine. Homes had been sold for trailers and RVs to live in throughout the process. Relationships were changed because a former spouse or partner could not accept the primary personal caregiver role. Older parents were pressed into assistance when younger children or siblings changed their minds.

"If we will be quiet and ready enough, we shall find compensation in every disappointment."
~ Henry David Thoreau

The *Primary Personal Caregiver's Guide* stated that you were to demonstrate the effort and ability to gain all the knowledge necessary to provide care for the patient during all phases of the transplant process. Besides the impossible situations the patients were living with by just trying to stay alive, they also had to contend with who would or would not be there for them.

Change-of-mind choices by initial caregivers are made all the time. In talking with numerous patients, I found some of the stories surrounding their situations pretty amazing. With huge disappointments within some families of people not taking on the roles of primary personal caregivers, there were also delighted surprises over the offers of those who came to the rescue.

Since we never really know what is going on in someone else's life, judging others is a fruitless act. Some of the responsibilities of the primary personal caregiver are absolutely daunting. There is the worry that one wrong move could lead to a life-threatening emergency. Oh, and by the way, there was a strong probability but no guarantee that the patient would survive.

For instance, I had to learn how to use a feeding

Chapter 6: Where Do We Go Now for This Transplant?

tube, load medications into special boxes and administer them. Fluids were given with varying degrees of thickeners, so Joe wouldn't aspirate. Water had to be sterilized. There was preparation of certain foods, recording vitals measurements and helping him with his swallowing exercises. I had to become familiar with a spirometer. There was so much to learn. These were more moments of, "You want me to what?"

I never wanted to become a nurse or a psychiatrist. My thoughts can scatter far and wide. I didn't think I could trust myself with prescribing specific doses of medication. Psychiatrists are medical doctors, psychologists are not. Having to keep track of details on a daily basis was a real energy drain. I would sometimes slip up on remembering my own heart meds. The thought of anyone else depending on me for intensive daily care ripped me up inside and out.

The risks of slip-ups for Joe were much greater than for me. I was feeling sheer terror. All I could think about was after Joe goes through all this, I'm probably going to kill him. I will give him the wrong medications, wrong doses, non-sterile fluids or foods, screw up the feeding tube, and everything else that I can do wrong.

I am a thoughts and emotions person. I am great at facilitating personal and professional growth and development with others. I have done that for many years. All this physical stuff is anathema to me. I found myself thinking that I would probably go to prison because no one would believe his death was an accident. They would say that as a professional, I should have been smart enough to know better. My ineptness and inadequacy haunted my many sleepless nights.

> *"We forget that life isn't as bad as we're making it out to be. We also forget that when we're blowing things out of proportion, we are the ones doing the blowing."*
> *~ Richard Carlson, PhD*

Happily, I can inform you now that none of this came to pass. Joe is now in almost two years of wonderful recovery following the operation. Much of that is due to his own excellent knowledge of his anatomy and physiology, as well as having a fantastic follow-up program with his transplant team.

What I learned:

This was a period of time during which I was pretty disgusted with myself. My self-pity parties only served up sour wine and stale cake crumbs. The balloons were all popped. Besides that, nobody came. From now on I'll call in a party planner. They couldn't be any worse.

Exercise:

Stop "shoulding" all over yourself. I really mean it. Stop it! Life isn't fair. It is just your time in the barrel. You did not write this script. You somehow showed up in it without even auditioning. Just play your part as best you can. Eventually this play will fold. At least you know you are not good at drama…or are you? Start directing your visualization to that great musical you will be starring in before you know it. There, now doesn't that feel better?

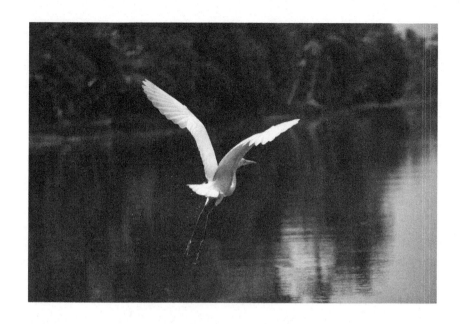

CHAPTER 7:

Is the Wizard of Oz Available?

A Heart, a Brain and Courage

"Start by doing what's necessary; then do what's possible; and suddenly you are doing the impossible."
~ Francis of Assisi

Let me say here that most of the care experience Joe and I received at Duke University Hospital was way above average. The expertise, helpfulness, courtesy, and genuine concern by so many from the top down were unlike any other hospital we had been to.

There were few really long waiting periods between appointments. Scheduling was done quickly and efficiently. The hospital is huge. It took weeks to learn how to get from point A to point B, C, D and E. Many people were helpful in guiding us through the maze. Smiles and random acts of kindness were offered everywhere.

Valet parking was expensive at $9 a day at least three times a week for almost a year. We had been surprised at the cost of the service at Duke Hospital. In Virginia when I spent months at the heart hospital in Norfolk, the service was free for cardiac patients and visiting disabled family members.

However, it was really necessary. First, the public parking garages were quite a hike to get to both the clinics and main hospital areas. Getting Joe in and out of the car with his oxygen tank and wheel chair and then hiking the long halls to his appointments was physically taxing.

Upon arrival at curbside parking, the valet drivers would get Joe into a hospital wheelchair and load his oxygen tank onto it. I didn't have to do this. I would turn over the car keys and then start pushing Joe to the first clinic appointment. There his personal tank could be changed out for one assigned to the hospital. Throughout a long day the hospital

Chapter 7: Is the Wizard of Oz Available?

tank could be swapped out for a fresh one. At the end of the day's sessions his personal tank would be loaded back onto the wheelchair and we would go to the lobby to await the delivery of our car. This often took a good while. However, the valet would help him get back into the car with his own oxygen tank fully in place.

For most of us we take breathing for granted. For Joe and others like him, his next breath depended on an oxygen supply source. It leaves a person in a fearful, helpless state. If that supply is cut off he will most surely die within a matter of minutes if he can't get emergency help. Can you imagine living like this?

After our drive home, I would pull out his own wheelchair, so he could get back inside the house. Sometimes we would arrive just as the next ten to fifteen oxygen tanks were being delivered. Both of us would usually take a nap and then get up to go over to the independent senior living center's dining room for dinner. We would return and finish the night out with watching the news and a couple of other TV programs. The next day the same pattern would all begin again.

Every weekday there would be more mandatory clinics. There were ongoing classes or the pre-op conditioning work. These involved blood draws, pulmonary tests, procedures and exercises, counseling and so on. This price had to be paid for Joe to stay in the program and to be ready when the lungs became available.

After four and a half long months of hard work, in April Joe was finally told he had been listed to receive the double-lung transplant. He had fulfilled the physical requirements to endure the transplant operation. At last the light of hope was rekindled. He was on a list with 17 other men and women in his rehab group. They all had different requirements. Their sizes, gender, age, blood types, length of lungs and type of lung deficiency and disease among other factors, affected where they were on the list.

THEN...on June 17 at 12:30 a.m., the phone call woke us. "We are harvesting a set of lungs for you right now. We need you here in 15 minutes!" Oh my God! It was happening! We threw our clothes on and were loaded up and in the car within seven minutes. We had driven the route to the hospital so many times that the car knew the way there. What was different and great was that at that hour there was little traffic, so I was able to drive at a pretty good clip. After all the months of driving this route, I had it down pat. There were two red traffic lights I paused at and then blew through. I figured that if a police car stopped us I could ask him to escort us the rest of the way to the hospital where the transplant team was waiting for Joe.

Duke offers a free parking service for accompanying family members of ambulance patients

Chapter 7: Is the Wizard of Oz Available?

heading to the Emergency Room. This was offered as well at the main hospital for transplant recipients headed to those operating rooms. I would have to say that it was clear that transplant cases were real VIPs at Duke. Whatever those teams wanted, they got.

As we approached the sign-in desk, a team member was already en route to get Joe to the operating rooms. I was able to go with him to the Pre-Op prep area. I sat in a corner and watched the systematic efficiency of several team members as they prepared him for the surgery. They used comforting words and emitted a calmness to put both of us at ease while they were doing their tasks. Ten minutes later I kissed him, and he was wheeled away to the O.R.

Now that was an odd moment. Within the last twenty minutes I had barely breathed. Everything was rapid movement forward. Now everything seemed to be at a complete stop for me. I stood there in the white fluorescent-lit hallway watching him being wheeled away and wondered if I would ever see him again alive. God only knows what he was thinking himself. This was about to be the biggest thing that ever happened to him in his life and he really didn't know how it was going to turn out either.

I was escorted to a comfortable waiting area. Not many people were there, and the lights were low in case people wanted to sleep. It was hours before dawn. I found a cozy corner area where I could spread out. A pillow and blanket were offered to me and I curled up with them. As I started to come down from my adrenaline high, I found myself wide awake and feeling numb. I didn't know how to feel. This had to be limbo...the in-between spiritual space.

> *"Faith is the bird that feels the light when the dawn is still dark."*
> *~ Rabindranaath Tagore*

I began to pray and eventually moved into meditation. I didn't feel anxious. Though it was around 2 a.m., I called Joe's son and daughter. I told them about all that had transpired so far and that I would keep them informed.

We were warned through our classes that sometimes patients had to go through "dry runs." This meant that something had gone wrong with the donor's lungs. The size could have been wrong upon initial inspection, or there was too much time between procedures that made the lungs less viable, or an infection could have been found that was not known about in the donor. There was a myriad of factors that all had to be satisfied before the actual transfer. If any of these were found, the patient was sent home to await the next possibility of a compatible donor. In Joe's rehab group of 18

Chapter 7: Is the Wizard of Oz Available?

listed people, several had this happen to them. As you can imagine it was disappointing and added to their stress.

Around 6 a.m. the surgeon came out to tell me that the first lung had been inserted successfully. No dry run here. Joe was in it to win it. Though probably not a good idea with your own family member, I would have loved to have been a fly on the wall of the operating room watching everything. It must be an amazing process to see. It gives me an excuse to continue to watch the TV show, *Grey's Anatomy*.

Finally, at 11 a.m., the surgeon returned to tell me the other lung transplant had also gone well. Feeling elated, I wanted to tell everyone I knew the good news. I chose, however, to only stay connected at that time with his children. It was still a fragile time of great vulnerability. I believed it would be best to wait until the team in the ICU gave us some more information. The next big hurdle was making sure he would not reject the new lungs. They were foreign materials in his body that had to be accepted.

I was allowed to come back to the ICU to see Joe around 2 p.m. He was heavily sedated and hooked up to what looked like every machine they had in the hospital. I was told that all the readings were looking good and he would be out for some time. His post-op ICU team was totally dedicated to him and he was being closely monitored. No one would leave him alone. I was given permission to go home and get some rest. About an hour later I did. After walking and feeding the dog and myself, I fell into bed and into a deep sleep. The past 16 hours had been a blur and I almost felt sedated myself.

When I returned to the hospital I walked into ICU and Joe was awake, on his feet and being helped in moving into the hall with a tall walker. My mouth dropped open in amazement. It had only been 24 hours since the transplant. How could this be? This was truly a miracle!

He was hooked up to a lot of medical instruments but his eyes were smiling as was the ICU team. They said that he was doing so well he would soon be able to leave ICU and be moved to another wing for the step-down recovery process. Wow! I was filling up with joy.

And then...and then...something went wrong. Joe's body was not rejecting the lungs but his former happier demeanor was changing. He started regressing. The upbeat attitude and mood suddenly became rather dark. He was being closely monitored but the team couldn't quite pinpoint where the actual problem was. Joe began to exhibit clinical paranoia. He believed everyone, including me, was trying to kill him. I had studied cases of it but had never seen a full-blown paranoia manifestation before.

Chapter 7: Is the Wizard of Oz Available?

The team had 24-hour "sitters" with him that I figured out were actually on suicide or another type of violence watch. After a lot of diligent teamwork, they found that Joe's body had developed an allergic reaction to one of the major anti-rejection drugs. This had manifested for him in the symptoms of paranoia. A different drug protocol was begun. A positive shift took place over the next couple of weeks. Joe's mood brightened. His healing now began to quickly move forward.

Through all of this I now had to make changes to my own daily routines. Part of the responsibilities of the primary personal caregiver was to be present every day at the hospital. I was usually there from 7:30 a.m. until 5:00 p.m. That way I could be present for each day's progress reports whenever the team members made their rounds. I also accompanied him as the wonderful nurses kept helping Joe advance with his rehab walking challenges. It kept his body moving and strengthening.

When a patient is assigned to a step-down recovery area it means they have to be "weaned off" of the constant acute critical care received in an ICU. The step-down process is the next step of recovery that eventually gets the patient out of the hospital and sometimes into rehab. Though care is still a steady and careful monitoring of the patient by highly skilled transplant medical staff, the patients are now on a ward with others.

I practically lived at the hospital for about a month. I would go home to tend to the dog, shower, grab a bite and drive on back. Unfortunately, the step-down area Joe had been randomly assigned to was in an older part of the hospital. The rooms were small and dreary. It made maintaining an upbeat attitude a bit of a stretch, but I tried. Though their first priority was Joe, the medical staff and transplant team were always courteous and kind and tried to be helpful to me. They regularly kept me informed of his physical status.

Joe's daughter was able to visit for three days and spend some time with her dad. Her presence was a good thing. He responded well to her and she wasn't among those he had thought were trying to kill him.

It was great to take two days off to spend with myself for the first time in forever. I was ecstatically grateful.

I spent both days with my fantastic furry friend. We had rescued Mystique 16 years before. She had been a four-month-old puppy who had been cast off by a family who had decided she would be too big for the small child they were raising. Boy, did they lose out.

She was an alpha female among other big dogs, except for Great Danes. She found their size really impressive. However, her gentle temperament and love for children and even other small dogs was special. I had seriously considered putting her into training as a therapy dog. Due to various circumstances and timing I was unable to proceed with that. She was definitely uplifting when she was brought in to see me during my own former stays in rehabs.

I didn't realize how therapeutic she would be as I travelled on my own odyssey. She was my Toto. Every day I had to return from the hospital to attend to her needs. She was the bright spot I looked forward to. Mystique was my touchstone to loving and being loved. She would allow me to bury my tears in her fur. Her big sloppy kisses would dissolve them as well.

On our walks I could enjoy her pleasure as she inspected and sniffed at so many things along the way. She seemed so delighted. The long days alone had been hard for her, too. Her doggie grins always lightened my state of mind. Every day, no matter how tired or low I was, Mystique was there to give me some comfort.

At certain places she would stop and look up at me to tell me this was where she wanted to roll in the grass and scratch her back. Before we had moved, she had a big back yard in which to do all that. In the last eight months, she had to adjust to that lack of freedom. Yet I still could feel her unconditional love and what seemed to be acceptance of the present situation.

"A dog has one aim in life... to bestow his heart."
- J.R. Ackerley

What I learned:

When a big battle is going on, a lot of trenches get dug. Sometimes you have to climb out of them for a rally. Other times you jump into them for a retreat. You may find buddies or strangers next to you in extremely vulnerable conditions like your own. You will get to know the pervasive smell of the dirt all around. Foul odors of all types can become part of the territory. What really matters is survival with honor. It is the best you can hope for. Oh, and it's good to have a War Dog with you.

Exercise:

I found that visualization of the outcomes I desired helped to lighten up my present moments. I could hold that brightness for only two minutes and I would feel the shift. My body would straighten and my breathing would even out. I would see the many beautiful gifts that were in my environments. For example, a sweet smile from a child, a pretty flower springing up from a crack in a sidewalk, or a neighbor sharing with me some of her big bouquet of flowers she had just brought home. My whole vibration would change. I could do this as often as I chose.

If I went back to just seeing negativity or feeling self-pity I would lose the energy, my shoulders would slump and I would miss the gifts of the moment.

Which experience would you want more of? Use your mind to control your moments. You are your own creator of your own experience.

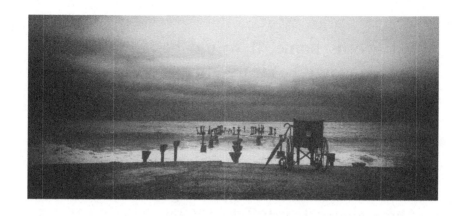

CHAPTER 8:

What Happens Once the Ruby Slippers Have Been Clicked?

"It's a thing to see when a boy comes home."
- John Steinbeck, The Grapes of Wrath

AT LAST, ON JULY 11, a month after the transplant and the daily intensive rehab, Joe was able to come home. He was walking and free from the constant hook up to an oxygen tank. The escort out of the hospital was the last wheelchair needed. The sun was shining, and he was breathing the air.

Hallelujah!

I drove us home. It would be about a month before Joe would be cleared to drive. His body had to adjust to being in new environments with new medications. His reaction times would be slower for a while. He even had to get used to being upright. He previously was all hunched over from continuous sitting and shallow breathing.

Once again, I didn't know how to feel. I was happy but not ecstatic. Our world was changing once again. What was the new normal? We had been so deep in the unhealthy normal that went before. Where were we now? We were quiet with each other. I was aware that as he was looking around on the trip home, he was experiencing the world in a new way. I was marveling at how straight he was sitting and without any paraphernalia on him.

When we arrived home, I drove into the garage. Joe got out and walked into the house on his own. This is when I started grinning. I took the wheelchair out of the trunk and left it folded up in the garage. We then folded up his other wheelchair and rollator that were propped against a dining room wall and put them out in the garage for donation. I felt my "happy meter" begin to rise further.

The oxygen condenser in his room was disconnected and moved into the dining room with the 15 tanks of oxygen and all the breathing hoses. The dispensing company was called to come and pick everything up.

Joe no longer needed to be attached to anything. He was free of trying to find enough strength to get into a wheelchair at night to get to the bathroom in time. He was even able to stand up in the shower again. He had meat on his bones and the ashy pallor was gone. Though he still had a ways to go with his recovery, the strength and health he now exhibited helped us both to begin to exhale. We would just sit and look at each other in awe over the miracle that had been given.

Like Dorothy when she was returned to her Kansas home, I was filled with gratitude. "There's no place like home," is the wish of coming back to what you have known. It usually signifies a safe and familiar place of normalcy. We didn't have that as yet, but we knew that we sure were a lot closer to it than we had been in years. We just had to re-establish what that was for us now.

There was a beautiful moment that took place at the independent senior living center that we will never forget. A few days after we had returned, Joe decided he wanted to go to the dining room for lunch and dinner. The administration staff greeted him with great warmth and generosity and then made an announcement to everyone that he had returned.

Now most of the residents, there were over 100, had seen what bad shape he was in for the seven months we had been there. When Joe walked into the dining room filled with over 50 people, the amazement and tears on their faces was an incredible sight to behold. He received a standing ovation and even the kitchen and maintenance employees were part of it. You kept hearing the word "miracle" everywhere. So many of them and their faith communities had been keeping us in prayer.

> *"God can restore what is broken and change it into something amazing. All you need is faith."*
> *~ Joel 2:25*

Full recovery without any form of rejection of the lungs became the main focus. A new post-transplant regimen at the rehab center began. It was still five times a week but the exercise period was for two rather than three hours. This was to help his body continue to recover from the trauma of the extensive surgical procedure of the transplant.

Joe steadily regained more strength and stability with the rehab team's help. The post-op groups served as a hopeful incentive to those struggling in the pre-transplant groups. They knew that this group had succeeded in doing the hard work the new ones were trying to do.

It was great to see the group continue to grow as more and more received their transplants. We would often run into other group members at the numerous follow-up clinic visits at the hospital. The physical changes that were taking place among them were sights to behold. When many of them greeted one another, you could see a deep level of appreciation that passed between them. No one else but another who had received this gift could fully understand what they had been through.

Sometimes we primary personal caregivers would also, with a smile, knowingly acknowledge this. There was also the below-the-surface understanding between us of our own journeys. The range of our caregiving was varied among us. Some had more people to help with it than did others. The financial cost was high for most of us. Yet now we could witness what it was all for. Yup, grins all around.

For me the greatest help I had was Joe himself. He had been a marathon bicyclist and a fencer. As an athlete, he knew his body extremely well. He was able to discover and redefine what his physical limitations were. To this day he is totally committed to his recovery.

Due to his extensive military training and expertise he was able to structure systems that supported his established goals. He kept precise records of everything including his medications and daily dosages. All of his appointments, contacts with phone numbers and transplant team names were also covered. The charts he made on his iPad were marveled at by his physicians, nurses and technicians.

Within a month he was off of liquid thickeners, sterilizing his own water and filling the special water containers. His appetite was increasing as well as his stamina. He never needed a feeding tube. Boy, was I grateful! I think I dreaded that the most. I guessed that I wasn't going to kill him after all.

We no longer needed valet parking either. We could pull right into a handicapped parking space in the hospital garage and Joe would walk to his appointments. It was good exercise for him and there were many benches in the halls if he needed to rest.

One day, as he had long wanted to do, Joe joined me on the daily walk with our dog. She kept looking around at him with wonder that he was there. Though Joe had to sit and rest after a little while, she and I continued on while Joe enjoyed the beautiful setting. He had never really seen the pretty lake with all the wildlife himself. I had just shared some pictures of it that I had taken.

Upon returning and seeing Joe a bit farther on, I dropped the leash and Mystique went bounding over to him with the pure elation only a dog can bestow on you. Yes, as you can already tell, I am a prejudiced dog lover. My heart was overflowing with joy as was Joe's. It was another deep moment of gratitude for the miracle of the gift of his new lungs.

"Too much of a good thing can be wonderful!"
~ Mae West

I don't know about you, but while I was in the throes of getting through the daily struggles I didn't often think about the imaginary donor. This transplant could only come about at the ultimate expense of another's life. I think there was a certain amount of depersonalization that was necessary to get to the point of the actual transplant procedure. I do remember, however, thinking about it as we were driving to the hospital shortly after midnight in June. Somewhere not long before, the donor had died. While we were experiencing some trepidation and a lot of hope, others were facing finality.

I was wondering how many other lives would be changed that night. Not just lungs were being harvested. Other organs for various patients were coming available as well, perhaps from the same person.

It reminds me of a story about a conversation that takes place between a chicken and a pig. The chicken talks about the effort she puts into being the provider for the farmer's daily breakfast eggs. The pig replies that he will provide a lot of tasty bacon to go with those eggs...but for him it's a one-time effort.

We will probably never know who the donor was without permission from both families. No contact can be made for a year following the transplant. Absolute confidentiality is paramount to this program. It is a good policy. The donor family needs time to mourn. The patient's body also needs time to adjust to the foreign matter within it. The risk of rejection takes time to decrease in probability. Knowing that somehow their loved one's organs had been used to help others live can be somewhat comforting to family members. Learning that the organs didn't help would only add to the grief.

The topic of organ transplants isn't one that usually comes up in most casual conversations. People usually have limited knowledge about them and there is an edge of morbidity to it. My personal experience on the topic before the situation with Joe had not been something I shared very often with others. It has a lot to do with which side of the process you are on.

Many years ago, I lost a son in a freak bicycle collision with another child's Big Wheel. The child ran into my little guy as he was coasting down a hill on his bike. Sean landed on his head on the sidewalk. It was right in front of our home. My son was five and a half years old. After three days in the hospital and surgery for brain injury, he passed. My husband at that time and I were asked if we would allow organs to be donated. I was so in shock that I couldn't bear to think of doing that. However, for some reason I did agree to allow his eyes to be donated. I was told a 22-year-old girl who was not much younger than me was given the ability to see with that gift. To this day, I am glad I did this. That girl's world, to literally be able to see it, was changed forever.

Young people think they are immortal, as I once did. If they are open, some may be convinced that putting organ donor on their licenses is the gift that keeps on giving. The second chance at life for millions of people has truly become a reality. Deaths of all types happen every day to people of all ages everywhere. However, the need for transplants always exceeds the number of organ donations available. I think anyone who becomes an organ donor is a real superhero and deserves a cape.

"Life doesn't give us purpose, we give life purpose."
~ The Flash

What I learned:

With every major life change comes deeper understanding with wisdom. It brings home Einstein's guidance as he said that we can't solve our problems with the same thinking we used when we created them. Every life change contains new properties, ideas, challenges. They may be similar to former ones in some ways but not all ways. We are not the same person going through them. Changes have taken place all along the way. When we apply an openness to what they are teaching us, we can be guided to new and often better solutions for the problems before us.

Exercise:

Think about a time when you had to go through another problematic situation earlier in your life. How did you solve that? How would you solve it now? What changed and why?

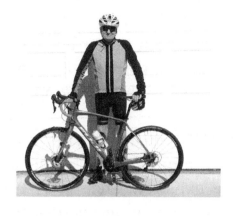

CHAPTER 9:

Are We There Yet?

The Wicked Witch Is Dead

*"The greatest achievement of the human spirit is
to live up to one's opportunities and
make the most of one's resources."*
~ Luc de Clapiers

I AM HAPPY TO say that everything slowly but surely has become much better. Joe's first purchase after his transplant was a brand new hi-tech bicycle and an indoor training system. To be able to ride a bike again had been a major incentive to keep struggling on in his pre-transplant program. The bike shop gave him a huge discount when they found he was returning to biking post-surgery. The owners wanted to make him a poster boy. They asked his permission to use him as part of a marketing campaign for a new store they were opening. The gift just kept on giving.

He has steadily advanced in the number of miles he can bike. There are good biking trails around us that he has explored. There have been a couple of setbacks, like becoming overheated, to let him know when he has over-taxed himself. I don't think I will ever be comfortable with him doing marathons again. I do think, however, that he is going to always be pretty protective of those new lungs. He won't be doing anything too rash that would compromise his anti-rejection protocol.

Joe's physicians marvel at how quickly his overall physical and cognitive recovery has been. For them, he is the shiny example of the results of their excellent lung-transplant program, especially at his age of 68. I wouldn't be surprised to read about his case in some medical journal.

He will be on many medications and strong anti-rejection drugs the rest of his life. There will be ongoing follow-ups no matter where we are. The team keeps close tabs on all these patients. We have met people who have lived for another 20 years or more following their lung transplants. This really is a second chance at a much longer life.

The first Christmas following Joe's surgery we were able to put up our Christmas tree that had

Chapter 9: Are We There Yet?

been packed away. Unfortunately, the box that held many of the Christmas ornaments that were special hand-made mementos from family members could not be found. This included my daughter's clay handprint at age five.

There was a whole Nativity set I had made in ceramics when I was in my twenties that was missing. Many of our beautifully designed annual White House ornaments were in that box as well. These and other ornaments from special friends would no longer hang on our tree.

I had packed that box protectively with two of my beautiful Flokati throw rugs. Old friends had brought the rugs back to me from Greece over 30 years ago. These had provided lovely décor to all of my homes since then. This box had evidently been moved by the movers into the wrong room during the sorting.

Since I hadn't unpacked these things during the prior December when we moved into our present home, nothing could now be done. The moving company searched their warehouse, but it was not in their inventory. They told us that the movers from that time no longer worked for them.

Even if the items had found their way into the estate sale inventory, most would have been sold or given away. Another farewell to the past.

I was disappointed for a few days but decided to get over it. This was a Christmas for gratitude, not regret. We still had other boxes of ornaments to use and new ones to signify and celebrate a new life for and with Joe. Besides, my daughter offered to make me a new ornament of her 40-plus-years hand.

Unfortunately, we lost our sweet dog Mystique a short time later. Her arthritis and old age (17) were the culprits. If it had been a year earlier, I honestly believe it would have seriously affected Joe's and my pre-transplant struggles. Caring for her gave us both further incentive to "keep on keepin' on." We still grieve over her and miss her with all our hearts. My walks around the lake without her have become easier with time. I greet the other dog walkers with a smile and sometimes a tear.

"If there are no dogs in Heaven, then when I die I want to go where they went."
~ Will Rogers

We took our first trip together about a year after the surgery. It was over a five-hour drive to Washington DC to visit with family members. There was a lot of driving between places while we were there as well, but Joe managed most of it. It gave him a new sense of independence again.

The best part was Joe being able to finally be with his grandsons and daughter. He was able to interact with them in ways that we couldn't have imagined even a year before. Trips to special museums and candy warehouses were highlights.

With this healthy physical progression there has been mental rehabilitation as well. One of the great activities here at the center has been a weekly senior discussion group called Socrates that was started several years ago. About 15 to 20 people attend including some local philosophy graduate students. Perhaps they feel they get a better chance to express their opinions here than with their own parents.

Current event topics are submitted from the group and voted on as to priority for discussion. It can get pretty lively. Joe serves as the group facilitator. He is adept at adding his extensive knowledge of American, military and world history to help with the blind spots of many topics. When I attend I am amazed at how rich his memory is again. The paranoid was once again the professor.

When we had first met, part of my attraction to Joe was that he was no mental midget. We had many interesting discussions over a vast array of subjects. We both enjoy the fact that our present community consists of people of many educational levels and cultures. Their idiosyncrasies add the color. We can learn something new every day. Even the gossip is juicy.

> *"There is no great genius without some touch of madness."*
> *~ Aristotle*

What I learned:

Trying on a new life with former favorite shoes doesn't always work. I used to wear high heels to my corporate job every day. Once I established my home business office I no longer had to do that. I often worked with my clients on the phone or web while wearing slippers or sandals. I often walked barefoot all over my house. Over time my feet spread to a half-size larger. I didn't realize it until I tried to wear the old heels. My feet were pushed forward into a smaller toe area. I was hobbled in no time. Baby needed a new pair of shoes!

Releasing the past can be like that. We can pretend nothing has changed until a new situation challenges us to be open to what the reality is now. Each decade that I have lived has brought me the need for a new pair of shoes. Part of that time we bring in all that we have learned and experienced from before. It seems to happen gradually, like my feet expansions, but then there is an awareness of the change. We are asked to make a choice to incorporate something new and move forward. I think I am a little quicker now with that awareness and far more accepting. My environment, relationships, career and even my wardrobe have "moved on."

At present, Joe and I are really enjoying each other again. I am far more relaxed and content in my surroundings. I am enjoying a renewal in both family relationships and friendships. I have a revitalized career focus. I have also been surprised at my enjoyment of a community I wouldn't initially have chosen. I like my new shoes.

Exercise:

Suppose today you were given $1,000. Now for some of you this would be a drop in your bucket. You will just reinvest it. For others it might be the price of an airline ticket to see an old friend who is not well. Maybe you will give yourself a spa monthly membership. How about several theater tickets? Maybe you'll keep it in your security box in case of an emergency.

Now ask yourself, how would you have spent this just five years ago? What has changed? Do you need a new pair of shoes?

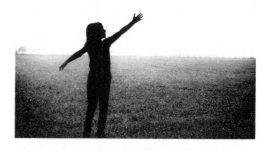

EPILOGUE:

Is That a Rainbow?

*"All you need is love.
But a little chocolate now and then doesn't hurt."
~Charles M. Schulz*

SO, AM I AT the end of my odyssey? Who knows. I would guess that at least for this leg of it, I am. The tension from fear and constant struggles is now greatly diminished. The exercises I offered to you are still helpful in my day-to-day living. I can breathe deeply and sleep well once more. A little melatonin here and there is still appreciated.

Joe has become quite self-sufficient for his self-care. Therefore, I have been able to look at future endeavors as real possibilities for my own life. I did learn to ask others for help. I hired both book-writing and business coaches. In the last nine months

I have written this book and co-authored another one on the topic of success. You can get a free copy of "Success Is Yours!" at my website:

www.drdonnamogan.com

I have also re-established my coaching business, Core Values Coaching, in a new state. Professionally my favorite thing to do is serve my clients through one-on-one and group coaching. They have come to me from all over the world. Knowing I am helping others transform and enhance their lives gives me a great sense of purpose with every coaching session.

I am back to developing new online-coaching programs. They had been tabled when I had to close my former business due to our severe medical issues. You can find some of these new programs at my website. I love the creativity that goes into playing with ideas and shaping them into helpful strategies and techniques for others to play with. I may even go back to doing some public speaking again.

Through this odyssey I have personally expanded my strengths, talents and wisdom with which to serve others. I now feel I am able to give my clients an even richer experience with my refined skills honed with new insights. Happily I am able to return to a venue that uses my own core values.

Beauty is one of them. It takes my breath away as I see Spirit shine through people, nature, and synchronicities. I witnessed profound beauty in ways others cared for not only the transplant patients but me as well. The random acts of kindness I found everywhere were often overwhelming. I think I became more consciously aware of them because my personal need was so great. It was the lengths that people went to in order to be of help that I found deeply beautiful.

I have a rather wicked sense of humor, another core value, and I am glad to be experiencing it again. Of all my natural gifts, this is one I truly treasure. I used to take it for granted. Now, however, I try to consciously use it in all kinds of situations. I set an intention each day to help lighten up at least one other person's day. Because of Joe's and my renewed relationship, there is a lot of love and laughter in our home. Laughter lets loose the endorphins for healing.

This odyssey can now be summed up in my mind as,

"Man makes plans... God laughs."
~ Old Rabbinic saying

"The most wasted of all days is one without laughter."
~ E. E Cummings

Taking things for granted, including your own natural talents, is a big mistake. Depression, fear and resentments cloud over the beautiful gifts each of us has within us. During the dark times, we can lose our sense of self-worth and self-confidence.

We can read in Psalm 30 that after the night endured, Joy comes with the morning. In other words, keep remembering that "this, too, shall pass." Once we see the light begin to come in, we usually go out to see what it is all about. I am happy to say it is all about everything.

Joy is ever present. Gratitude allows you to see it. Appreciation takes it right into your heart to savor it. This is a gift that is always being given and can keep on giving. It just takes practice and continually developing conscious awareness.

When we put our whole selves consciously into the present in a receptive mode, we receive the present…it is the gift/present. Here we are not divided by illusionary thoughts around what is over with or hasn't yet happened. The present is where we are fully available to receive beauty, wisdom, understanding, friendship, joy, surprise, comfort, and love. We have the freedom in each moment to select and accept that moment's gift…or not. It is our choice as to what we focus upon.

Yes, life really can be good again.

Made in the USA
Las Vegas, NV
02 April 2022